Anti-Cancer Nutrients: Fucoidan & AHCC

What You Need To Know About Fucoidan & AHCC. Understand Their Benefits And Side Effects For Cancer Treatment

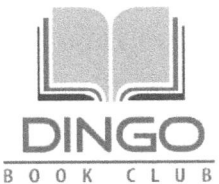

DINGO
BOOK CLUB

"Great Books Change Life"

© **Copyright 2018 by Dingo Publishing - All rights reserved.**

The contents of this book may not be reproduced, duplicated or transmitted without direct written permission from the author.

Under no circumstances will any legal responsibility or blame be held against the publisher for any reparation, damages, or monetary loss due to the information herein, either directly or indirectly.

Legal Notice:

You cannot amend, distribute, sell, use, quote or paraphrase any part or the content within this book without the consent of the author.

Disclaimer Notice:

Please note the information contained within this document is for educational and entertainment purposes only. No warranties of any kind are expressed or implied. Readers acknowledge that the author is not engaging in the rendering of legal, financial, medical or professional advice. Please consult a licensed professional before attempting any techniques outlined in this book.

By reading this document, the reader agrees that under no circumstances are is the author responsible for any losses, direct or indirect, which are incurred as a result of the use of information contained within this document, including, but not limited to, —errors, omissions, or inaccuracies.

Table of Contents

INTRODUCTION 5

CHAPTER 1: FUCOIDAN 7
    WHAT IS FUCOIDAN? 7
    HISTORY OF FUCOIDAN 9
    HOW DOES FUCOIDAN WORK? 10
    WHAT ARE THE CONVENTIONAL CANCER TREATMENTS? 11
        Surgery 12
        Radiation therapy 12
        Chemotherapy 13
    WHY FUCOIDAN FOR CANCER? 14

CHAPTER 2: BENEFITS OF FUCOIDAN 16
    ANTI-CANCER BENEFITS OF FUCOIDAN 16
    FUCOIDAN AGAINST FATIGUE 19
    FUCOIDAN AND CARDIAC HEALTH 19
    FUCOIDAN AND WEIGHT LOSS 20
    ANTI-AGING BENEFITS 20
    OTHER HEALTH BENEFITS 21
    USES OF FUCOIDAN 22
    SIDE EFFECTS OF FUCOIDAN 24

CHAPTER 3: AHCC (ACTIVE HEXOSE CORRELATED COMPOUND) 26
    WHAT IS AHCC? 27
    HISTORY OF AHCC 27
    HOW DOES IT WORK? 28
    BASIC CATEGORIES OF IMMUNITY 29
        Innate immunity 29
        Adaptive immunity 30
    WHAT DOES AHCC DO? 31
    MODIFICATION OF THE IMMUNE RESPONSE 32
    AHCC AND ITS BENEFITS 32
    ANTI-CANCER BENEFITS OF AHCC 33
    SIDE EFFECTS OF AHCC 34

CHAPTER 4: FUCOIDAN AND AHCC 35

- COMBINED EFFECTS OF AHCC AND FUCOIDAN 36
- BATTLE AGAINST THE SIDE EFFECTS OF STANDARD CANCER TREATMENT 37
- LIVER PROTECTION 39
- NUTRITIONAL ALTERNATIVES FOR BETTER LIVER FUNCTION 40
- DIFFERENT MECHANISM FOR IMMUNE SYSTEM STIMULATION 42
- HEPATITIS, SYMPTOMS AND ITS EFFECTS 43
  - *Symptoms:* 44
- COMMON TREATMENT PROTOCOL 45
- NUTRITIONAL INGREDIENTS TO FIGHT HEPATITIS 45
- FUCOIDAN AND ITS EFFECT ON THE VIRUS 46
- AHCC (ACTIVE HEXOSE CORRELATED COMPOUND) AND ITS EFFECT ON HEPATITIS 47

CHAPTER 5: FUCOIDAN AND AHCC SUPPLEMENTS 50

- RECOMMENDED DOSAGE OF THE SUPPLEMENTS 50
- SELECTING THE BEST HIGH QUALITY SUPPLEMENTS 51
- BEST SUPPLEMENTS IN THE MARKET 53
- WHERE TO BUY? 54
  - *Nature Medic Fucoidan powered with AHCC* 54
  - *Umi No Shizuku* 54

CHAPTER 6: PREVENTION IS BETTER THAN CURE 55

- SIMPLE WAYS TO PREVENT CANCER 56

CONCLUSION 62

BEFORE YOU GO 64

BONUS #1 69

BONUS #2 86

Introduction

I want to thank you and congratulate you for purchasing the book, "Fucoidan and AHCC – Anti-cancer ingredients".

Cancer is the most deadly disease, which affects millions of people every year across the world. With the increasing rise in awareness, many of us try to implement a combination of healthy diet and proper physical activity to keep ourselves away from the risk of cancer. We do come across cancer victims who are bravely facing the treatment and battling the disease. Apart from medicines and surgery, chemotherapy is an important treatment given to the people who are affected by cancer to help them cure the disease. These treatments are mostly painful for the patients and can affect their physical and mental strength.

Active Hexose Correlated Compound (AHCC) and Fucoidan are the two natural ingredients that help the cancer victims to strengthen the immunity when they undergo their treatment for cancer. Active Hexose Correlated Compound (AHCC), in its natural form, is used as a dietary supplement for general health purpose.

This book will discuss in detail about Fucoidan and AHCC (Active Hexose Correlated Compound), their brief history, their benefits on health and its uses, the different ways it helps by supporting the human body to battle those cancerous cells, its importance in medical field and their side-effects (if any).

I hope this book will help you understand what Fucoidan and AHCC (Active Hexose Correlated Compound) are and how it can help the cancer patients while undergoing their regular dose of treatment. We have tried our best to make the details simple for everyone to understand and I sincerely hope this book serves its purpose. Thanks once again for purchasing the book.

I hope this book serves as an informative and interesting read for you! Thanks again for purchasing this book. I hope you enjoy it!

Chapter 1: Fucoidan

Fucoidan, which is found in the cell walls of most species of brown seaweed, is a natural ingredient that carries with it all the healthy benefits of the sea life. They are known for strengthening the immune system of the body from blood clots, damage caused by chemotherapy and radiotherapy, osteoarthritis, viral infections, kidney and liver diseases. They can activate the stem cells and help in blocking the growth of cancer cells.

Apart from helping in cancer treatments, it fights fatigue, helps in weight loss and promotes cardiac health.

What is Fucoidan?

Fucoidan, which occurs naturally in the cell walls of brown seaweed, protects the plant from environmental challenges and waterborne pathogens. Fucoidan comprises highly complicated complex polysaccharides. They are generally found in different species of brown algae such as bladderwrack, Kombu, Hijiki, mozuku and wakame. Sea Cucumber, an animal species, also contains a form of Fucoidan.

Fucoidan has many different types of simple sugars that are linked to complex matrix with sulfate as the key component. Fucoidan is often referred as "sulfated polysaccharide". Fucoidan has a fundamental sugar subunit called Fucose, which is widely found on the cell surfaces of humans and a few other mammals. It is also found in plants, insects, mushroom, kelp (type of brown seaweed), etc.

There are two different forms of Fucoidan:

- F-Fucoidan (Composition is less than 95%)
- U-Fucoidan (has about 20% glucuronic acid)

History of Fucoidan

For thousands of years, most of the Asian countries had seaweed as their staple food. They were also used for treating inflammation, nausea, congestion, high BP (blood pressure), bacterial and viral infections, abscesses and tumors. Most of these seaweeds contain Fucoidan, which is the major "ingredient" that helped their therapeutic and dietary properties.

Though the history of seaweeds as 'medicinal agents' appears thousands of years ago, it was only in the twentieth century; fucoidan was recognized for its therapeutic properties, due to its natural ability of regulating the substances involved in cell growth and acting as NK (natural killer) cells.

Seaweeds were a staple diet for the people in the island of Okinawa (now part of Japan). Their cuisine was completely based on fucoidan rich seaweeds, which were consumed raw, used for garnishing, boiled for soup stock, etc. Since the island was located in a remote place, their unique dietary habits weren't open to the world until it caught the attention of researchers studying 'aging' in the twentieth century. They found that the island had some of the longest living humans in the world despite their lack of modern medical technologies. It was finally discovered that fucoidan - the slimy ingredient of seaweed was the reason behind their secret of long life and almost NIL or much fewer cancer victims. However, one needs to understand that not all fucoidans are the same. The class of natural compounds that exert beneficial bioactivities for human health criterion is completely dependent on the method of extraction and the seaweed species it has been derived from.

These fucoidan extracts are used in dietary supplements, veterinary products, topical formulations for skincare or dermatology and a few medical devices.

How does Fucoidan work?

Fucoidan is very effective in mobilizing the stem cells and moving them to the place in the body where there is a need to replace the existing affected cells.

To be more specific, stem cells can actually transform the different kinds of living cells and also replace the cells that cause the cellular damage. Fucoidan can amplify specific kinds of stem cells and rescue the aging or old stem cells that act as pillars for reforming the inner walls of the affected blood vessels.

What are the conventional cancer treatments?

Does Fucoidan fight against the cancerous cells directly? To answer this question, we need to understand how cancer is usually treated. Most of the cancer treatment involves chemotherapy (treating using chemical substances like cytotoxic or other drugs) and radiotherapy (treating using some form of radiation or X-rays). When the cancer patient is treated using these methods, the cancerous cells are destroyed by these rays or chemical drugs which can also affect the other living cells required for our body's regular functions. Let us have an elaborate discussion on these treatments and their side effects.

Based on the type of cancer and the patient's medical condition, cancer is treated in many different ways. There are three conventional methods for cancer treatment and they are:

a) Surgery

b) Radiation therapy

c) Chemotherapy (including immunotherapy and angiogenesis inhibitors)

(a) Surgery

Surgery, often performed along with radiation therapy or chemotherapy, is done to remove the tumors or "as much cancerous tissues as possible". Based on the stage of the cancer, the treatment and diagnosis for the same is done. There are also instances when the cancerous tissues or the tumors cannot be removed and in such cases to reduce the pain or dysfunction caused, palliative surgery is performed on the patient. This surgery can remove the masses causing the pain or disfigurement or intestinal obstruction. Palliative surgery doesn't cure the cancer or prolong life but is done mainly to lessen the discomfort caused to the cancer victims.

(b) Radiation therapy

Radiation therapy is used to eliminate the cancer cells or shrink the tumors using certain type of radiation. This damages the cancer cells completely giving it no chance to multiply as the cells die due to high sensitive radiation. There are chances that it can cause damage to healthy cells. This treatment can be combined with surgery or chemotherapy or can be given alone based on the 'stage of the cancer'.

(c) Chemotherapy

Chemotherapy affects the entire body as it targets rapidly multiplying cancer cells. Since our body contains lot of other cells that multiply at larger rates, like the gut cells and hair follicle cells, it causes side effects like stomach upset or hair loss or vomiting or nausea. Chemotherapy can be performed via IV rays or as pills. Depending on the stage of cancer, chemotherapy can be given with the use of angiogenesis inhibitors or immunotherapy.

There are cancerous tumors, which create new blood vessels and increase the blood supply to the tumor allowing it to grow at rapid speed. Angiogenesis inhibitors prevent the growth of these new blood vessels and are used to treat colon, breast, lung, rectum, kidney cancers and brain tumors.

Immunotherapy or BRM (biological response modifiers) or biotherapy effectively increases the immune response of the body to cancer by working on the white blood cells or WBC with no effect or little effect on the healthy cells.

Why Fucoidan for cancer?

Fucoidan does have numerous effects against different kinds of cancer. It regulates the vital molecules that force the destruction of the tumor cells and also slows the vascular tissue formation, which feeds the tumor growth. It also acts as anti-cancer chemotherapeutic agents, which means combination of fucoidan and chemotherapy at lower dosages will reduce the toxic effects.

Fucoidan is highly recommended for having these three anti-cancer abilities:

- Ability to instigate Apoptosis
- Enhancing the body's immune system
- Suppressing Angiogenesis

Destruction of cells from 'within' by activating the digestive enzymes contained in the cells is called apoptosis. It is a form of 'cellular suicide'. Apoptosis limits the tumor development as it destroys the cells by forcing the cell to kill itself using the digestive enzymes contained in the cell. Fucoidan, which is an ingredient given to mankind by nature, can instigate apoptosis in cancerous cells thereby disrupting and killing the mitochondria (energy membrane) of the cancer cell. The best part is – Fucoidans cytotoxic effects only targets the cancer cells and does no damage to the healthy cells.

Fucoidan enhances the body's immune system by triggering the immune mechanism of the intestines and by stimulating the immune cells of the gut (abdominal region).

Fucoidan also blocks the formation of new blood vessels that can accompany the growth of infectious tissues in tumors leading to cancer. The best way to attack cancerous cells is to completely cut off the supply of blood to the tumor and Fucoidan, which is a natural "angiogenesis inhibitor", fulfills this.

When Fucoidan is used along with the conventional cancer treatments in an efficient way, it makes the entire process more powerful and effective.

Chapter 2: Benefits of Fucoidan

Fucoidan causes certain types of cancer cells to self-destruct without affecting the normal cells. It also strengthens the immune system, enhances anti-pathogenic responses and reduces allergic reactions. It has extensive health benefits on the body as an antioxidant, reduces blood lipids, acts as an antivirus, anti-inflammatory, anti-tumor, anticoagulation agent and also works on gastrointestinal protection.

Anti-cancer benefits of Fucoidan

Fucoidan has strong anti-cancer properties that include cancer inhibition, pathogen inhibition and immune modulation. It is the best oral supplement therapy, which can be used along with chemo or radiotherapy.

The most common anti-cancer benefits of fucoidan are:

- It enhances antitumor effects

- It is actively used in treatments for breast cancer, liver cancer, colon cancer, lung cancer and prostate cancer.
- It down-regulates the pancreatic cancer cells
- It reduces the side-effects of chemotherapy
- It strengthens immune system
- It works on neuroprotective actions
- It blocks cancer cells from developing and growing
- It improves blood circulation

Fucoidan caused stomach, lymphoma, colorectal cancer cells and leukemia to destruct on their own at a research conducted in the Biomedical Research laboratories. It was also proved by the Institute of Research of Glycotechnology Advancement that U-fucoidan could successfully destroy the number of rapid growing cancer cells.

Fucoidan helps the body with required nourishment to boost the natural production of adult stem cells in bone marrow; which means the body's ability to heal and repair the injured tissues increases due to the adult stem cells, which circulate in the blood. The surprising factor is that it doesn't contribute to abnormal cell growth (tumors or cancers) even with its ability to encourage cell regeneration.

The ability to simulate natural killer cells plays an important role in destroying virus-infected cells thereby increasing the immunity in the body.

Fucoidan against fatigue

Fatigue is found to be dangerous for the body as it reduces the individual energy resources of the person. It has a cynical impact on the bone density of the cancer therapy and also affects the individual's nutritional condition of the individual. Studies have proved that more than 30% of the chemotherapy patients undergo fatigue and around 60% of the colorectal cancer patients are affected by grade 2 and grade 3 fatigues.

Fatigue is usually treated by using antidepressants. A clinical research confirmed that the cancer patients who were administered with Fucoidan supplements were able to go through the pain of prolonged chemotherapy sessions without fatigue.

Fucoidan and cardiac health

The International Journal of Biological Macromolecules published their findings in June 2012 and confirmed that Fucoidan is beneficial for the cardiac health. An individual can save himself from heart muscle injuries like heart strain, heart attack, etc by taking regular fucoidan-rich food or a fucoidan supplement.

Fucoidan and weight loss

South Korea published their research on "fat-fighting properties of fucoidan" in the 2011 issue of "Marine Drugs". The research showed that fucoidan can help in stimulation of lipolysis (the breakdown of fats and lipids by hydrolysis to release the fatty acids), which means that this ingredient can work wonders in treating and preventing obesity.

Anti-aging benefits

The most interesting benefit of this natural substance is its role in activating a vital enzyme which influences lifespan thereby enhancing the anti-aging benefit. The key enzyme is the sirtuin 6, which plays a major role in influencing the different range of cellular functions in the human body.

This particular enzyme is good for age-associated diseases like metabolic syndrome, obesity, insulin resistant type 2 diabetes and chronic inflammation. Fucoidan is the only polysaccharide to simulate sirtuin 6.

Other health benefits

Apart from acting as an anti-cancer nutrient, Fucoidan is also used for other health benefits and acts as a dietary supplement.

- It helps reduce inflammation in organs like kidney, liver and heart, as it possesses genetic anti-inflammatory effects.
- HCV-related chronic Hepatitis C virus infection can be treated using Fucoidan as it reduces the HCV RNA levels significantly.
- It helps reduce liver fat, limit diabetes-induced liver disease & kidney damage and helps treat non-alcoholic liver disease caused by pathogen.
- It also works on protecting the brain function by reducing or reversing brain aging and disease.
- It shows inhibitory effects on Herpes, HIV and Influenza
- It helps by preventing hair loss by strengthening the hair and promoting its growth.
- Fucoidan helps to treat hypertension or high blood pressure

- It treats allergies, bacterial, viral infections and inflammations
- Bladderwrack (type of brown seaweed) helps in treating wounds and prevents infections
- Kelp (type of brown seaweed) helps in treating common colds, influenza, herpes, etc
- Bladderwrack also helps in treating hypothyroidism (due to the high iodine content) as well as gastrointestinal disorders (constipation, indigestion, gastritis)
- The bioactive component in Fucoidan, which modulates and reduces the activity of digestive enzymes helps in shedding weight faster.

Uses of Fucoidan

Fucoidan has many uses to ensure we maintain a healthy body with strong immune systems.

- Fucoidan is helpful for people suffering from osteoarthritis (pain or stiffness in hip, thumb joints and knee) and when the fucoidan extracts are consumed orally, osteoarthritis is significantly reduced.

- One of the techniques to treat "surgical adhesions" uses fucoidan and turns out to be effective. A surgical adhesion (tissues and organs sticking together) is a fibrotic reaction caused by inflammation.
- Fucoidan works effectively and improves liver functioning when toxins or pathogens enter the liver.
- Fucoidan compounds have a retarding effect against blood coagulation (blood changing to solid or semisolid state).
- Fucoidan provides neural-protection and is quite essential for the proper functioning of the brain.
- Based on a study conducted in 2008, fucoidan extracts have shown inhibitory effects on few viruses especially against herpes simplex virus infection by causing hindrance to the growth of the specific virus

Side effects of Fucoidan

No major adverse side effects have been reported from using Fucoidan but there are relatively few potential side effects. The side effects are more specific to the type of Fucoidan extract used, as a particular type of seaweed can be more harmful compared to another one.

- If you are taking blood-thinning medication while consuming Fucoidan, you could have increased risk of bleeding
- The high amount of iodine in brown seaweed (kelp or bladderwrack) can give thyroid problems if consumed in excess.
- There might be chances of toxic reaction due to arsenic if the brown seaweed is taken from contaminated waters.
- Temporary diarrhea, which disappears after continuous usage, is the most common side effect for high dosage, especially when used as supplement.
- If you experience bloating, the fiber in fucoidan could be the reason as the component is a dietary fiber.
- Apart from the sugar content 'Fucose', it may also contain sugars like xylose or

- mannose (depending on the type of brown seaweed), which can cause diarrhea.
- If you are allergic to soy, you may also face allergic reaction on Fucoidan consumption. Allergic symptoms may include heavy breathing, swelling in the face and throat, increased heart rate and hives on the skin.
- If you have low blood pressure, it is best to avoid Fucoidan or consult your physician for the right dosage before taking the supplements.
- Mozuku (Fucoidan extract) has blood thickening quality, which might not be good for people with high blood pressure.

Though Fucoidan has more benefits compared to the side effects, one should understand that it couldn't be used as a replacement to proper medical therapy but only as an aide to the conventional cancer treatment. If you plan to take this extract as a regular supplement, it is advisable to get the consent of your physician.

Chapter 3: AHCC (Active Hexose Correlated Compound)

In medical industry, antibodies, immune system substances, cytokines and vaccines are synthesized in the laboratory to be used for cancer treatment. These are called Biological Response Modifiers (BRMs). Similar to Fucoidan, AHCC is one such BRM. It makes an attempt to strengthen or reinstate the body's ability to fight the sickness by changing the body's immune defence interaction with the cancer cells.

AHCC has been successful in treating quite a range of health conditions, from the minor health issues such as cold, flu and influenza to the major deadly diseases like diabetes, cancer, hepatitis and cardiovascular disease. A human body's compromised immunity leads to these acute and chronic conditions and AHCC boosts one's natural immune response thereby helping the body to fight the foreign threats.

What is AHCC?

Active Hexose Correlated Compound (AHCC) is an alpha-starch rich nutritional extract from Japanese Shiitake mushrooms, which are known for their healing properties for centuries. It is an enzyme fermented extract of the mushroom, which is used as dietary supplement.

Active Hexose Correlated Compound (AHCC) is used along with conventional cancer treatments, as it is the strongest known immune strengthening BRM according to Japan. The general public of Japan and China use AHCC as a supplement for acute infections and normal health maintenance. They don't need a prescription and is termed as "functional food" legally. It is promoted for immune support and hence commercially available.

History of AHCC

In 1987, the University Of Tokyo Faculty Of Pharmaceutical Sciences combined with other researchers and developed AHCC (Active Hexose Correlated Compound) to be a natural product, which can help in regulating high blood pressure. It is majorly known for its potential to stimulate the immune system as it protects the body against infections, cancers and viruses.

It has been used as natural supplement along with the treatment of patients diagnosed with cancer, diabetes, hypertension, AIDS, hepatitis C and few other autoimmune diseases. A few claim to have used it for treating wounds, fatigue syndrome, stomach ulcers, gum diseases and multiple sclerosis.

How does it work?

The presence of cancer cells and tumors are uncovered throughout the body by a healthy immune system using the process called "immune surveillance". Cancer cells have the ability to hide, thereby avoiding the detection by the immune system and this is where "immune surveillance" plays a crucial role. When the immune surveillance is restored, the tumor cells are unmasked allowing the body's immune structure to detect and destroy them again.

Researchers tried to find out if AHCC (Active Hexose Correlated Compound) can help the effort of "immune surveillance" and the result was positive. AHCC reduced the formation of melanoma (tumor of melanin forming cells) and reduced the tumor size. They significantly increased the levels of tumor antigen-specific immune cells. It was proven that AHCC enhances tumor immune surveillance by regulating both cell-mediated and humoral responses.

Basic categories of immunity

Human body has two basic categories of immunity:

- Innate immunity (Body's first line of defense)
- Adaptive immunity (Body's second line of defense)

(a) Innate immunity

Your body's innate immunity attacks immediately without a second thought against the threat without any specifics. The key players in the first line of defense are:

- Dendritic cells (these are white cells that present the foreign elements to B and T cells)
- NK cells or the natural killer cells (white blood cells injects granules into the abnormal or infected cells forcing them to explode)
- Macrophages (white blood cells absorbs the cellular remains and bacteria by engulfing them)
- Cytokines (the chemical messengers which makes the immune cells to coordinate a response when it communicates)

(b) Adaptive immunity

Your body's adaptive immunity creates a distinct response to a specific microbe. The key players in the second line of defense are:

B and T cells (Lymphocytes has the capability to recognize the prior invaders and ruin them with a particular response; B cells develop in bone marrow while T cells develop in thymus)

What does AHCC do?

Active Hexose Correlated Compound (AHCC) has anti-inflammatory and antioxidant effects that can enhance the response of the body's immune system.

- It supports immune health by increasing the natural killer cell (NK cells) activity and enhances the effects of killer T-cells and cytokines.
- It reduces C-reactive protein (CRP), as it is anti-inflammatory resulting in minimal health risks of unresolved inflammatory processes.
- It helps to recognize the tumors and cancer cells by increasing the immune system's ability.
- It protects the immune system from chemotherapy side effects and strengthens the effect of chemotherapy treatment
- It protects liver and its functions
- It guards against bacterial and viral infections
- It prevents metastasis

Modification of the immune response

It has been proved in clinical trials that AHCC (Active Hexose Correlated Compound) modifies the innate and adaptive immune response by increasing the:

- Production of cytokines
- Number of dendritic cells
- Number of T-cells by 200%
- Activity of NK cells by 300 – 800%
- Doubling the population of macrophages (in certain cases)

AHCC and its benefits

Active Hexose Correlated Compound (AHCC) is available as dietary supplements and it carries numerous benefits for the normal crowd. Check out the benefits here:

- AHCC can minimize the side-effects such as vomiting, weight loss, decreased liver functions, etc., during the chemotherapy and radiation treatment sessions
- AHCC helps get rid of viral infections like flu and also prevents the same when taken along with the flu shot.

- It acts as a BRM (biological response modifier) which protects the liver from damage, increases the survival chances of patients affected by liver cancer and reduces viral load of hepatitis patients
- It strengthens the cellular immunity in healthy humans

Anti-cancer benefits of AHCC

The following are proved anti-cancer benefits when AHCC (Active Hexose Correlated Compound) is used along with the conventional cancer treatment.

- It helps in recurrent ovarian cancer treatment
- It enhances and strengthens anticancer / antitumor effects
- It down-regulates the pancreatic cancer cells
- The side effects caused by chemotherapy like neutropenia can be reduced
- It actively promotes immune response
- It increases the survival options and improves the outcome of the medical treatment of patients affected by advanced liver cancer.

AHCC (Active Hexose Correlated Compound) produced from fermented medicinal mushrooms has proved to increase the production of the body's NK (natural killer) cells to support the immune system. The NK cells or natural killer cells destroy the abnormal cells and foreign organisms in the body. It cannot be referred as a cure but merely considered as a supplement to support the other drugs used in the treatment process for best effective results.

Side effects of AHCC

AHCC (Active Hexose Correlated Compound) has never shown any reported side effects when taken as supplements with conventional medicines or when taken in appropriate amounts. Loads of patients have benefitted while AHCC has been included in their treatment.

When AHCC (Active Hexose Correlated Compound) underwent a clinical trial (phase 1) in 2007 with 26 healthy human test subjects aged between 18 and 61, it was concluded that around 85% of the subjects could tolerate the mild adverse side effects and hence, AHCC was declared as a safe supplement in clinical practice and the side effects are very mild and tolerable.

The most common complaints could be diarrhea, bloating and nausea, while some may experience fatigue, headache and foot cramps if AHCC is consumed in liquid form.

Chapter 4: Fucoidan and AHCC

The last three chapters would have given a clear picture on what Fucoidan and AHCC (Active Hexose Correlated Compound) are and the benefits they bring to the health condition of the human body. Both Fucoidan and AHCC have been proven to act as a natural complementary medicine for cancer treatment.

AHCC (Active Hexose Correlated Compound) is used in 700 plus hospitals and clinics in Japan while the US National Library of medicine published close to 600 Fucoidan related researches. Both these components are used against most cancers and tumor treatment; and help boost body immunity for chemotherapy and radiotherapy patients.

These natural extracts show favorable benefits to people who are suffering from various forms and severity of cancer or tumor, by effectively killing the cancer cells without causing damage to the other living cells.

Combined effects of AHCC and Fucoidan

Let us understand how the combination of AHCC (Active Hexose Correlated Compound) and Fucoidan is helpful in completely eliminating the cancerous cells or by having an increased chance in reducing the cancerous cells completely. It also works on the various side effects triggered by the conventional treatment.

Fucoidan and AHCC (Active Hexose Correlated Compound) form the best combination to prevent cancer and treat the cancer if it has already attacked the human body. With more people wanting to try evidence based alternatives and high-quality complementary therapies, it is proven that AHCC and Fucoidan blend is the best medical combination of the many available. This perfectly balanced blend can provide extraordinary health benefits in its natural form when it combines the brown seaweed extracts and specially fermented mushrooms in the right measure.

Fucoidan promotes stimulation of the immune gut cells, angiogenesis suppression and apoptosis induction while AHCC (Active Hexose Correlated Compound) supports the functions of Fucoidan by enhancing the function of the liver by using immune system modulation via white blood cell activation. When these two components are combined together, they act as a support system for the conventional cancer treatments and helps in maintaining a healthy Qualify of Life (QoL) for the patients to pursue their treatments further.

Battle against the side effects of standard cancer treatment

Cancer develops due to different factors such as lack of physical activity and proper nutritional diet; having a weak immune structure that is not able to kill the cancer or tumor cells on an average scale. On top of that, when your body is exposed to a bunch of dangerous components like radiation, toxins, etc, it further increases the cancer cell development at an abnormally high level without being able to be sustained by the body's immune system. It is therefore considered important to enhance the immune system to prevent cancer or battle against it, particularly if you are already undergoing treatments that are weakening your immune function.

When you consume several substances like AHCC (Active Hexose Correlated Compound) and Fucoidan under certain circumstances, the combined effect of the components can help boost the immunity and support the immune system to reclaim equilibrium in a more efficient and effective way. Oncologists are very much aware that the cancer patients will need their immune structure to be boosted to enable the body to build up the immune system for fighting off the cancerous cells and prevent medicines or strong radiations from reducing the effect of the body's natural defenses. To stop the cancer affecting every other living cell in the body, it is vital to have a strong immune system.

Combining Active Hexose Correlated Compound (AHCC) and Fucoidan to the conventional cancer treatment in the people helps the body to strengthen its immune system to help attack the cancer cells. This strengthened immunity system will help in reducing the side effects of the anti-carcinogenic agents and improve the therapeutic effects.

In the worst-case scenario, if the cancer treatments (surgery, radiation therapy and chemotherapy) are unable to cure the tumor, then the patients should be open and free to seek other modes of treatment too. It has been clinically proven that, by providing the patients with Active Hexose Correlated Compound (AHCC) and Fucoidan, the immune system is strengthened and enhanced, which results in the body tolerating the side-effects and maintaining a better QoL (quality of life), thereby helping them to pursue their treatments further.

Liver Protection

The health condition of advanced cancer patients are extremely weak with the damaged or unbalanced internal organ functioning as these patients would have already undergone treatment processes like chemotherapy, radiotherapy or surgery for a few months. The liver is one of the most important organs among the others to get affected during the process.

The liver has many important functions in our body like processing the food, drugs, toxins, producing bile to help in food digestion, filtering blood and having protein added to the blood, etc. If the cancer is located in the liver or starts spreading the cancerous cells to the liver, it can damage the function of the liver as the tumors can infiltrate the tissues and vessels surrounding the organ and make it extremely difficult to remove the tumor. When there is liver failure, the body shows specific changes like developing jaundice or abdominal girth, which is the accumulation of fluid in the abdomen thereby, causing vomiting and nausea.

So it is vital to maintain a liver that is strong enough to have a steady functioning of detoxification taking place thereby helping the body to restore the energy it requires. Though Fucoidan is best for supporting the liver in its detoxification process, AHCC (Active

Hexose Correlated Compound) would be the best alternative as studies have proved that AHCC is effectual in stimulating the liver functioning better.

Nutritional alternatives for better liver function

Liver cirrhosis is the most common and dangerous problem. Cirrhosis is the disfiguring of the liver (liver scarring), which stops the liver function when scar tissue blocks the blood and the bile flow to the liver. When a foreign body attacks the liver, the organ gets damaged as the cells are destroyed as a scar tissue formation occurs. This process is called Fibrosis. When the liver completely hardens and shrinks as it gets scarred, it leads to cirrhosis and the damage cannot be rectified. Heavy drinking, viruses (Hepatitis C or B), diabetes, environmental poisons, autoimmune hepatitis (process of the liver getting attacked by our own immune system) thinking it to be a foreign body), certain over-the-counter medicines, etc can cause cirrhosis.

Maintaining a well balanced diet with the right combination of fats, proteins, carbohydrates and adequate calories is very important for liver-affected patients to help in liver cells regeneration.

Combination of AHCC (Active Hexose Correlated Compound), Agaricus blazei (a type of mushroom species) and Fucoidan can help in bringing back proper functioning of the liver.

The Journal of Gastroenterology and Hepatology - published the following results:

"Fucoidan causes anti-fibrogenesis in liver-induced cirrhosis through the down-regulation of transforming factor 'beta 1' and 'chemokine ligand 12' expressions, and that scavenging lipid peroxidation is well-incorporated in the liver."

There was also another research published in the Cancer Chemotherapy Pharmacology Journal showed that there has been considerable improvement in the function of the liver cirrhosis patients who had advanced hepatocellular carcinoma when they were administered with AHCC (Active Hexose Correlated Compound).

Agaricus blazei, a mushroom variety from Brazil, was used for medicinal purposes (without the need of prescription) widely. This medicinal mushroom repairs the damage caused in the liver when used in combination with AHCC (Active Hexose Correlated Compound) and Fucoidan.

All these researches proved that, with medical management, proper diet and combination of the nutritional ingredients (AHCC (Active Hexose Correlated Compound), Fucoidan and Agaricus blazei), the progressive rate of liver damage can be actively slowed down.

Different Mechanism for immune system stimulation

Fucoidan and AHCC (Active Hexose Correlated Compound) can stimulate the immune system by two different methods:

1. By activating the white blood cells (WBC)
2. By stimulating the gut immune cells

White Blood Cells activation by Active Hexose Correlated Compound (AHCC)

Active Hexose Correlated Compound (AHCC) modulates the cell-mediated immunity by forcing the activation of the lymphocytes and WBCs which in turn attacks the abnormal cells, external viral or bacterial pathogens or the virus infected cells which try to enter the body. AHCC doesn't directly destroy the cancer cells but battles against it indirectly by stimulation of the immune-competent cells and securing the body's natural response.

Gut immune cells stimulation by Fucoidan

Fucoidan has high molecular weight that enables it to get easily digested in the gut when the body recognizes it as a foreign component. Fucoidan can also enter into the central portion of the small intestine when detected by the TLR receptor. TLR receptor is a class of protein that plays an important role in the innate immune system. When these receptors are activated, they induce signal events that help in regulating the immune mediators' expression.

Fucoidan can also influence the cell-mediated and innate immunity by interacting with T-cells, monocytes, lymphocytes and macrophages. This can strengthen the host's response to the immune system to diseases like cancer, which are chronic to the body.

Hepatitis, symptoms and its effects

Hepatitis is a violent disease, which attacks the body like 'sleeper cells'. This virus spreads and primarily targets the liver to keep 'itself' reproducing and latches to one's body like a parasite. When the immune system attacks the virus, it slows down and hides in various other body parts and waits to strike back again when the person's immune system grows weaker. Since the virus conceals in other parts of the body, a liver transplantation will not help but will enable the virus to restart its vicious cycle with the healthy liver. Hepatitis C is the worst while Hepatitis A and B can be completely eliminated as long as the victim takes good care of his body.

Symptoms:

The body will start showing the symptoms within 5 weeks of the virus infection that can be acute or chronic.

Acute symptoms (short-term) would be pain in the liver, vomiting, nausea, fatigue, diarrhea, irritability, headaches, confusion, dark colored urine and grey/clay colored stools.

Chronic symptoms (long-term) would be liver cirrhosis, jaundice, fluid retention, chronic fatigue, itchy skin, weight loss, blood vomiting, hallucinations, and sleep disturbance and hepatic encephalopathy.

Additional symptoms (as discovered by traditional Chinese medicines) are vision problems, dry & brittle hair, discolored or pale fingernail beds, cramping, cognitive problems (not able to plan or think properly), disturbed sleep, hypertension, dizziness, joint issues, night blindness, piercing pain in the chest, tumors, irregular menstrual cycles, red eyes, trembling hands and feet, etc.

Common treatment protocol

Hepatitis ('Hepato' – liver and 'itis' – inflammation) is a viral attack on the liver leading to serious inflammation and few extreme complications. It is often said that 80% hepatitis infected victims do not show any symptoms of the disease whereas 20% of the hepatitis infected victims show problematic symptoms as the virus has the tendency to conceal itself in other body parts when it senses an external attack.

The first protocol for treating hepatitis would be to strengthen the victim's overall immune system to help in forcing the virus to get into 'hibernation mode'. It is a wonderful start to actual recovery. Often it is believed that researchers turn to holistic medicinal approach or ancient Chinese medicine for effective treatment of hepatitis.

Nutritional ingredients to fight Hepatitis

Fucoidan and AHCC (Active Hexose Correlated Compound) are mostly recommended to help in massive health improvement as they provide the body with initial support in taking the attack against the virus to one level above.

Fucoidan and its effect on the virus

HCV (Hepatitis C Virus) is an extremely violent virus which is dangerous and distressing to the liver and its severe infection can lead to liver cirrhosis which in turn causes liver cancer.

The researchers in Japan evaluated the antiviral function of Fucoidan on Hepatitis and published the following result:

"Fucoidan dose-dependently inhibited the expression of HCV replicon. At 8-10 mo. of treatment with fucoidan, HCV RNA levels were significantly lower relative to the baseline. The same treatment also tended to lower serum alanine aminotransferase levels, and the latter correlated with HCV RNA levels. However, the improved laboratory tests did not translate into significant clinical improvement. Fucoidan had no serious adverse effects."

It was concluded that Fucoidan is extremely safe and can display useful effects while treating people who are affected by HCV-related chronic liver diseases.

AHCC (Active Hexose Correlated Compound) and its effect on Hepatitis

AHCC (Active Hexose Correlated Compound), the natural compound, is recognized for its capability to increase the function of NK cells (natural killer cells) by 300% or more, and simultaneously simulating the macrophage, T-cells, and cytokine activity. This immune stimulation acts effectively with patients who have weak immune systems, which often lead to catastrophic ailments like hepatitis.

In few cases of liver cancer and hepatitis, the doctors have reported a good improvement in decreasing or eliminating the virus concentration in the blood, loss of platelets and stopping the deterioration of liver function after the administration of Active Hexose Correlated Compound (AHCC) to the patients.

Outcome of various case studies:

1) 3gms of AHCC (Active Hexose Correlated Compound) regularly on chronic hepatitis B patients had the following result:
   "Decline in the value of HBe antigens and increase in HBe antibody value"

   HBe antigen value stipulates the amount of hepatitis B virus and HBe antigen is the antigen that helps in eliminating the hepatitis B virus.

Initially the platelet count of the patient started decreasing but didn't continue to decline. Finally it was confirmed that hepatitis B virus was completely eliminated.

2) 3-6gms of AHCC (Active Hexose Correlated Compound) regularly used on hepatitis C patients resulted in the following:
"Considerable reduction in the liver enzyme levels and the 'loads' of other chronic diseases"

3) Continuous consumption of AHCC (Active Hexose Correlated Compound) for six months had shown around reduction of viral load by 80 percent.
Continuous consumption of AHCC (Active Hexose Correlated Compound) for twelve months helped in reaching the required viral load range in a few patients.

The studies also suggested having the following healthy recommendation would considerably help the body to cope with the attack:

- Balanced diet comprising of berries, nuts, vegetables and fruits.
- Sunlight
- Turmeric or curcumin
- Zinc supplements
- 3000 mg of Vitamin C per day
- Flax seed mixed with dairy-free yogurt
- Regular exercise (light)
- Sea salt (moderate usage on everything you consume)
- Small amounts of Selenium
- Dandelion
- Licorice roots

After numerous clinical trials and researches, it has been proven that Fucoidan can be effective for treatment of chronic diseases such as cancer and hepatitis, and is more advantageous when it is combined with Active Hexose Correlated Compound (AHCC).

Chapter 5:
Fucoidan and AHCC Supplements

We need to ensure that our health holds the top priority in our life. Natural supplements are always the best choice when it comes to making the best out of what is consumed into our body. It is an additional bonus when these natural extracts not only provide innumerable health benefits with recommended dosage but also ensures there are no adverse side effects.

Recommended Dosage of the supplements

The dosage of Fucoidan and AHCC supplements can vary based on the medical history but generally, the dosage amount is as follows:

- 1-2 gms of Fucoidan extract for general health benefits

- 3-6 gms of Fucoidan extract for cancer or other malignant diseases (as per the doctor's instruction)

- 3gms of AHCC a day for 28 days improves specific innate immunity (for general health benefits).

Have two capsules a day as a dietary supplement.

U-Fn Fucoidan capsules are effective for fighting cancer in the reproductive system, lower gastrointestinal tract and the blood when taken for 3-4 months.

Most of the Fucoidan supplements are powered with Active Hexose Correlated Compound (AHCC) and has a concentration of 85% and above.

Selecting the best high quality supplements

The best quality of Fucoidan comes from wakame-Mekabu (Undaria pinnatifida) and the brown algae mozuku (Cladosiphon okamuranus).

Ensure the following are strictly taken care of when you choose your brand:

- Mekabu and Mozuku are the only two kinds of Fucoidan used for dietary supplements
- The concentration should be higher than 85%

- They should have zero contamination and completely free from heavy metals or radiations
- Always select 100% natural or organic sources
- They should comply with Current Good Manufacturing Practices (CGMPs) and proper quality control
- Go for capsules which have only vegetarian ingredients (100% vegetarian)
- It is important that the right amount of the supplement is consumed.

The species 'Mozuku' which has the highest production of Fucoidan is cultivated mainly in Okinawa (Japan) while the other species 'Wakame' is found commonly in Australia, Argentina, China, Korea and Japan. After the earthquake and tsunami that shook Japan in 2011, the farming of brown seaweed (wakame) was affected in higher level due to increased radiation. It not only affected the locals who consumed seaweed as their food but also took a toll on the fucoidan dietary supplements.

It is always recommended to select 100% organic natural resources.

Best supplements in the market

Did you know that 1 kg of brown seaweed is needed to obtain 1 gm of Fucoidan? It is better to consume the extract supplements instead of eating 1- 2 kg of brown seaweed daily.

The following are the best two dietary supplements based on an independent research.

- Nature Medic Fucoidan with AHCC
- Fucoidan Umi No Shizuku

Nature Medic Fucoidan powered with AHCC combines AHCC mushroom extract with Fucoidan brown seaweed to formulate the natural dietary supplement with high quality control in Japan. This product contains organic Mekabu Fucoidan (from Australia) and Mozuku Fucoidan (from Okinawa, Japan) along with the Japanese Shiitake mushroom extract.

Umi No Shizuku uses the mozuku seaweed found in the waters of Okinawa, Japan in its purest form. This product also contains the properties of the Agaricus blazei mushroom mycelia extract along with the brown seaweed and this combination helps in boosting the body's immune function.

Where to buy?

Both the above-mentioned dietary supplements can be purchased online in Amazon.com after reading the user testimonials.

Nature Medic Fucoidan powered with AHCC

Amazon link:

- https://www.amazon.com/gp/product/B00MEXE96C

Umi No Shizuku

Amazon link:

- https://www.amazon.com/gp/product/B003LT6T3E

Chapter 6:
Prevention Is Better Than Cure

All said and done, it is better to give the necessary precautions required for the human body to develop its natural immune system and ward off these deadly diseases even before they penetrate into your body cells. Most of the time it so happens that these deadly diseases especially cancer would have found its way into your body because of the negligence one would have shown to it. It is important to understand your body, analyze the visible changes and take preventive measures before the bomb explodes on your head.

Not all cancer can be prevented but there some that can be, because most of the time, cancer is caused by unhealthy food choice, lack of physical activity and external factors such as tobacco, alcohol, infectious organisms, etc. There are a few which are caused by internal factors such as immune condition, inherited genetic mutations and hormones. It is necessary to consult your physician in case you belong to a family with a history of cancer or other medical issues that might lead to tumors.

Simple ways to prevent cancer

Let us look at the simple ways to prevent cancer and ward off any chances of the cancer cells to crawl into our body

- **Strict NO to sugary drinks and soda**
  Both sugary drinks and soda contribute to diabetes and obesity, which may increase the risk of endometrial cancer.

- **Add resistant start to regular diet**
  Green bananas, white beans and regular oats contain resistant starch, which can reduce the risk of colon cancer.

- **More standing and less sitting**
  Studies have suggested that people spending most of the day "sitting without much physical exercise" have 24%higher risk of colon and endometrial cancer. Take regular breaks and walk around. Make a conscious effort to stand whenever possible.

- **Eat broccoli once or twice in a week**
  Steamed broccoli contains glucosinolate and is considered as a cancer-preventing food. Avoid micro waved or fried broccoli.

- **Wake up your body cells with sunlight**
  Vitamin D is an important energy source that is required for your body and close to 90% of the Vitamin D comes from the sunlight directly. People with Vitamin D deficiency have higher risk of breast, colon, ovarian, stomach and prostate cancer. Fifteen minutes of sunlight exposure to your body regularly can do wonders.

- **Add Kiwi to your fruit platter**
  Kiwi is packed with rich cancer-fighting antioxidants including lutein, copper, vitamin C and Vitamin E.

- **Safe sex**
  It is always advisable to have safe sex to reduce the risk of contracting HPV or human papillomavirus, as they can cause vaginal, penile, cervical and anal cancer.

- **Ensure you have a healthy weight**
  It is well known that obesity increases the risk factor of developing breast cancer. It is important to exercise regularly to burn the fat, which produces estrogen (known cause of breast cancer)

- **Don't drink too much alcohol**
  Women who drink one or two alcohol per day on a regular basis will have 10-20% greater risk of breast cancer

- **Tobacco is injurious to health**
  Regular smoking causes cancer in larynx, esophagus, throat, mouth, bladder, stomach, pancreas, kidney, cervix, bladder and lungs.

- **Say NO to consumption of animal products**
  Animal fats (meat and butter) is associated with increased risk of prostate cancer

- **Excess gluten consumption is dangerous**
  Wheat is the primary source of gluten as it turns into sugar in your bloodstream, which can feed cancer cells. It might affect your immune system making your body vulnerable to cancer cells.

- **Have a check on your calories**
  Avoid consuming calorie rich foods like chips, candies, dried cereals, processed food, etc on a regular basis.

- **Balance body fat and blood sugar naturally**
  Eliminate refined sugars and sweets from your diet and add fruits like berries, grapes or apples to your food bowl.

- **Regular medical check-up**
  Try getting a regular medical check-up once or twice a year to know your body condition. Earlier detection of ailment is always better.

- **Know your body**
  Self analyze your body once a while and consult a doctor if you come across sudden lumps or unexplained bleeding in your body.

- **Eat selenium-rich food**
  This mineral fights a variety of cancers and is a powerful antioxidant found in Brazil nuts, garlic, broccoli, pumpkin seeds and whole grains. Studies were conducted on prostate,

colorectal and lung cancer patients and it was proven that administration of selenium on them had reduced 67%, 58% and 45% of the respective cancers.

- **Add soy to your diet**
  Soy foods contain isoflavones, which regulates the body to respond to estrogens produced naturally. Soy intake has also reduced the number of deaths from prostate cancer and also has lower rates of breast cancer victims.

- **More fiber intake**
  35 gms of fiber each day reduces the risk of breast, mouth, ovarian, pharynx, rectum, stomach, prostate and colon cancers

Try taking a conscious effort in listening to your body and its needs. Anti-cancer foods, healthy lifestyle, the right choice of supplements like Fucoidan and AHCC, handling stress, etc can help you to lead a happy and healthy lifestyle.

Can you help me?

If you enjoyed this book, then we really appreciate it if you would post a short review on Amazon. We read all the reviews and your feedbacks will help us improve our future books.

If you want to leave a private feedback, please email your feedback to: feedback@dingopublishing.com

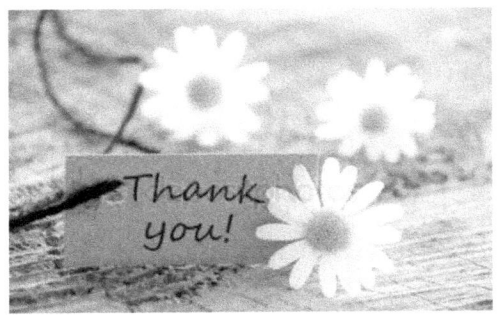

Thanks for your support!

Now, let's continue on next page

Conclusion

We have reached the end of this book. I hope the book was informative and simple to understand, as we have tried our level best to make it as simple as possible for an easy and interesting read. I would once again like to thank you for purchasing this book.

This book would have given an overview about Fucoidan and AHCC (Active Hexose Correlated Compound), its individual history, its role in cancer treatment and the necessity of having these anti-cancer ingredients to our diet. We have covered the primary objective of the book, which is to give the readers an idea about "the necessity of understanding the details of natural supplements used along with conventional medical treatments".

This book would also give a detailed description of the advantages a human body can have when both Fucoidan and AHCC (Active Hexose Correlated Compound) is used as a combined blend along with conventional treatments and also as a natural dietary supplement.

Treat your body with utmost care and boost your immune system by not giving it an option to make way for unwanted infection or diseases. Choose the right dietary natural supplement and consume them regularly post your physician's advice. Be aware of cancer and the different ways it can affect the body's organ. Constant vigilance and proper research can always be a blessing.

I sincerely hope that this book was useful and has helped answer most of the queries you had in your mind. My best wishes to you to lead a healthy cancer-free life. I hope that this book helps you with all the necessary information for you to share with the cancer survivors, especially if they are your near and dear ones.

Before you go

We have a surprise for you!

As a way of saying thanks for your purchase, I'm offering a special gift that's exclusive to my readers.

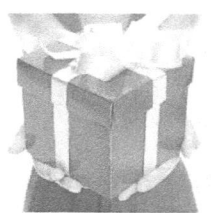

http://bit.ly/VBonus1

Another surprise! There are free sample chapters of our **best-selling** books at the end.

- Anti – inflammatory Diet for beginners by Jonathan Smith. (Page 69)

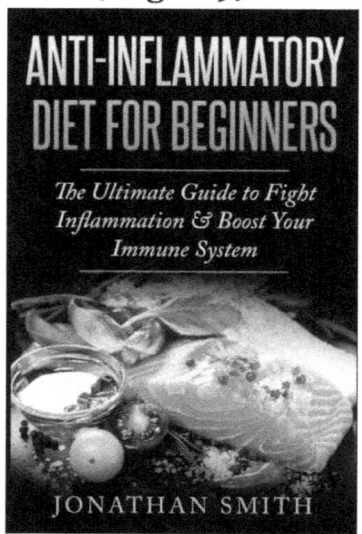

- Anti – cancer Diet by Olivia Green (Page 86)

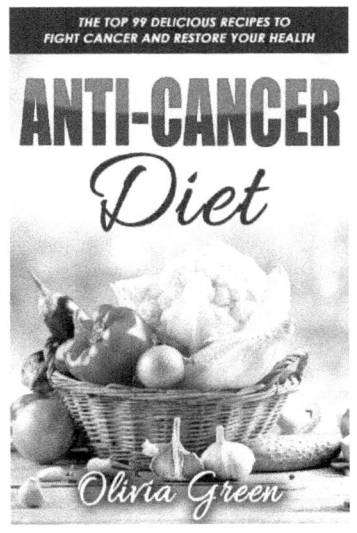

MORE BOOKS FROM US

Chia Seeds Cookbook

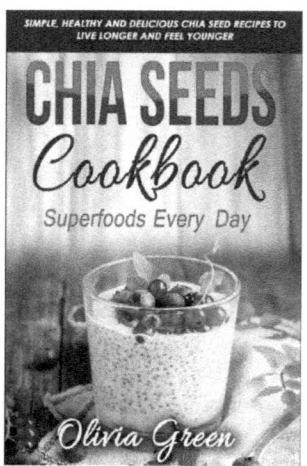

Kale Cookbook

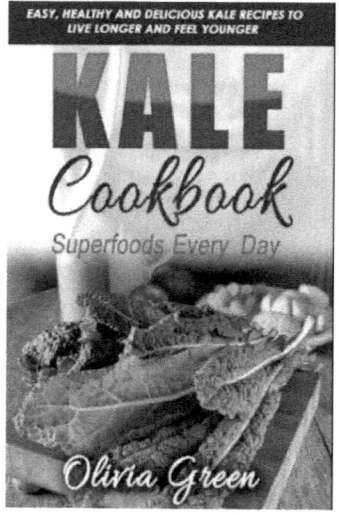

Intermittent Fasting by Jonathan Smith

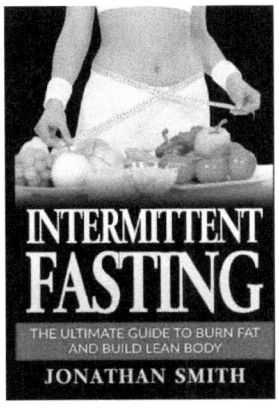

HIIT – High Intensity Interval training by Joshua King

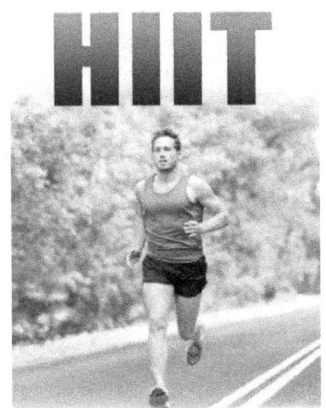

Procrastination by J. Martin

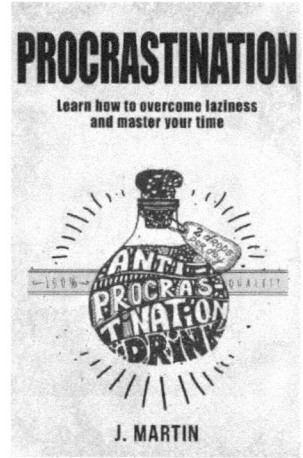

Accelerated learning by Jason Clark

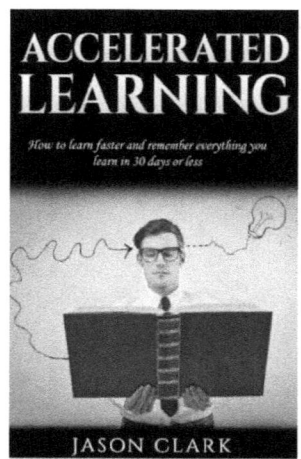

Bonus #1

Sample chapters of 'Anti – inflammatory Diet for beginners by Jonathan Smith'

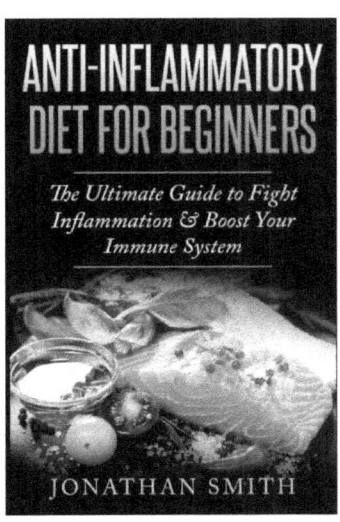

Chapter 1: Introduction to Anti-Inflammatory Diet

To make this book easy to read and follow, we will start by understanding inflammation and the anti-inflammatory diet.

In its simplest terms, an anti-inflammatory diet simply refers to a collection of foods that have the ability to fight off chronic inflammation in your body.

So what exactly is chronic inflammation?

Well, before we discuss that, let's start by understanding what inflammation is first.

So what is inflammation?

Inflammation is simply a term used to refer to your body's response to infection, injuries, imbalance, or irritation with the response being swelling, soreness, heat, or loss of body function. It is the body's first line of defence against bacteria, viruses and various other ailments. The goal is to 'quarantine' the area and bring about healing/relief. This is the good inflammation, as it is helpful to your body. It is often referred to as acute inflammation. However, there are times when the inflammatory process might not work as expected resulting to a cascade of activities that could ultimately result to cell and tissue damage especially if it takes place over a prolonged period. This is what's referred to as chronic inflammation. This type of inflammation has nothing to do with injuries; it is not as a result of an injury or anything related to bacteria, virus or any other microbe. And unlike acute inflammation that comes with soreness, pain, heat and swelling, chronic inflammation comes with another set of symptoms some of which include diarrhoea, skin outbreaks, congestion, dry eyes, headaches, loss of joint function and many others. This inflammation is what you need to fight using an anti-inflammatory diet because if it is not addressed early, it might result to a number of various chronic health complications that we will discuss in a while.

So how exactly does this chronic inflammation develop that would actually require a diet to undo? Here is how:

It all starts in the gut. The gut essentially has a large semi-porous lining, which tends to fluctuate depending on various chemicals that it comes into contact with. For instance, if exposed to cortisol, a hormone that is high when you are stressed, the lining becomes more permeable. The lining also becomes a lot more permeable depending on the changing levels of thyroid hormones. This increased permeability increases the likelihood of viruses, bacteria, yeast, toxins and various digested foods passing through the intestines to get into the bloodstream, a phenomenon referred to as leaky gut syndrome (LGS). The thing is, if this (the intestinal lining becomes damaged repetitively), the microvilli in the gut start getting crippled such that they cannot do their job well i.e. processing and using nutrients with some enzymes that are effective for proper digestion. This essentially makes your digestive system weaker a phenomenon that results to poor absorption of nutrients. If foreign substances find their way into the bloodstream through the wrong channels, this results to an immune response that could result to inflammation and allergic reactions. This form of inflammation can bring about different harmful complications. What's worse is that as inflammation increases, the body keeps on producing more white blood cells to fight off the foreign bodies that have found their way into the bloodstream. This can go on for a long time resulting to malfunctioning of different organs, nerves, joints, muscles, and connective tissues.

Chronic inflammation is harmful to your body and your brain. Let me explain more of this:

Your body is responsible for supplying glucose to your brain so that your brain can perform optimally. When you eat too much inflammation-causing foods, your body slows down its process of transporting glucose to the brain since it concentrates on fighting off the inflammation. Your brain then keeps asking the body for glucose since it is not getting its fill. This effect causes you to crave sugary and pro-inflammatory foods. Inflammation can also result to abnormal levels of water retention along with other problems that contribute to stubborn weight gain. This just worsens the condition and causes your inflammation to worsen. Unfortunately, majorities of dieters focused on weight loss only focus on reducing calories and fatty foods but pay very little attention to how eating pro-inflammatory foods may be contributing to an inability to lose weight quickly.

If inflammation persists, it can bring about a wide array of health complications some of which include:

- Obesity and chronic weight gain
- Lupus
- Arthritis
- Cancer
- Diabetes
- Celiac disease
- Crohn's disease
- Heart disease

So how exactly does inflammation lead to disease? That's what we will discuss next.

How Inflammation Could Lead to Diseases

It is possible to have a disease-free body, but only if you can manage to keep your body balanced. Diseases develop only when something upsets the equilibrium (balance) of the body. An abnormal composition of blood and nymph is a typical example of such imbalance. These two are responsible for supplying the tissues with nutrients and carrying away eliminated toxins, metabolic by-products and wastes from the liver and kidneys. When you consume unhealthy meals, it may affect the balance of blood and nymph in the body and lead to inadequate supply of nutrients and thus, the body would be unable to give adequate support to kidney and liver function. The consequence of this is that it exposes the body to the risks of several diseases and inflammatory conditions, which I mentioned earlier.

Food Allergies, Food Intolerance, and the Anti-Inflammatory Diet

Food allergies happen when your immune system reacts to the proteins in certain foods. Your immune system releases histamines that may cause production of throat mucous, runny nose, watery eyes, and in severe cases, diarrhea, hives, and anaphylaxis.

Your immune system's reaction to food allergies is to trigger inflammatory responses because when a food causes allergic reaction, it stimulates the production of antibodies that bind to the foods and may cross-react with the normal tissues in your body.

One of the highpoints of the anti-inflammatory diet is that it calls for the elimination of foods that promote allergies and intolerance.

How the Anti-Inflammatory Diet Works

To cure and stop incessant inflammation, you must eliminate the irritation and infection, and correct hormonal imbalance by eating specific foods while avoiding others. This would help stop the destruction of cells and hyperactive response of your immune system. When on an anti-inflammatory diet, most of the foods you shall be eating have powerful antioxidants that can help prevent and eliminate symptoms of inflammation.

For instance, anti-inflammatory foods such as avocados contain Glutathione, a powerful antioxidant. Radishes contain Indol-3-Carbinol (13C), which increases the flow of blood to injured areas. Pomegranates have polyphenols that stop the enzyme reactions the body uses to trigger inflammation. Shiitake Mushrooms are high in polyphenols that protect the liver cells from damage. Ginger has hormones that help ease inflammation pain.

We will discuss more on the foods you should eat and those you should avoid later.

In the next chapter, we shall look at the basic rules of the anti-inflammatory diet as well as how to get the best out of the diet program.

Chapter 2:
Basic Rules of the Anti-Inflammatory Diet

As is the case with any diet, the anti-inflammatory diet has basic rules but as you are about to find out, these rules are very easy to follow and straightforward: no extreme rules that would leave you cravings-crazy and running back to a poor eating style after a few days.

When following this diet, there are about 11 rules you should follow:

1st: You Must Eat at Least 25 Grams of Fiber Daily

These should be whole grain fibrous foods such as oatmeal and barley, vegetables such as eggplant, onions, and okra, and fruits like blueberries and bananas. These fiber-rich foods have naturally occurring phytonutrients that help fight inflammation.

2nd: Eat at Least Nine Servings of Fruits and Vegetables Daily

A serving of fruit refers to half a cup of fruits while a serving of vegetable refers to a cup of leafy green vegetables. You could also add some herbs and spices such as ginger, cinnamon, and turmeric, foods that have strong anti-inflammatory and antioxidant properties.

3rd: Eat at Least Four Servings of Crucifers and Alliums Every Week

Crucifers refer to vegetables such as Brussels sprouts, Broccoli, mustard greens, Cabbage, and Cauliflower. Alliums refer to onions, garlic, scallions, and leek. These foods have strong anti-inflammatory properties and may even lower risks of cancer. You should eat at least four servings of these every day, and at least one clove of garlic daily.

4th: Consume Only 10% of Saturated Fat Daily

The average daily recommended calories for adults is about 2,000 calories every day. This means you have to limit your daily saturated fat caloric intake to no more than 200 calories. If you consume less than 2,000 calories daily, you have to reduce accordingly.

Saturated fats include foods like hydrogenated and partially hydrogenated oils, pork, desserts and baked goods, sausages, fried chicken and full fat diary. Saturated fats often contain toxic compounds that promote inflammation, which is why you need to eliminate these foods from your diet.

5th: Eat a Lot of Omega-3 Fatty Acid Rich Foods

Omega-3 fatty acids rich foods such as walnuts, kidney, navy and soybeans, flaxseed, sardines, salmon, herring, oysters, mackerel and anchovies are an essential part of this diet thanks to their strong anti-inflammatory properties.

6th: Eat Fish Thrice Weekly

It is important that you eat cold-water fish and low-fat fish at least three times a week because fishes are rich sources of healthy fats and can be great substitutes for saturated and unhealthy fats.

7th: Use Healthier Oils

The fact that you have to reduce your intake of some types of fat does not mean you should stop consuming all fats. You only need to reduce or even eliminate the consumption of unhealthy ones and limit your intake of healthy ones like expeller pressed canola, sunflower and safflower oil, and virgin olive oil. These oils have anti-oxidant properties that help detoxify the body.

8th: Eat Healthy Snacks at Least Twice Daily

Unlike in most diets, in this diet, you get to eat snacks as long as it is healthy. You can snack on healthy foods such Greek Yoghurt, almonds, celery sticks, pistachios, and carrots.

9th: Reduce Consumption of Processed Foods and Refined Sugars

Reducing your intake of artificial sweeteners and refined sugars can help alleviate insulin resistance and lower risks of blood pressure. It may also help reduce uric acid levels in your body. Having too much uric acid in your body may lead to gout, kidney stones, and even cancer. A high level of uric acid in the body is usually because of poor kidney function. Overloading your kidneys with pro-inflammatory foods may reduce kidney function and subsequently lead to excessive uric acid levels in the body.

Reducing your consumption of refined sugars and foods high in sodium can help reduce inflammation caused by excess uric acid within the body.

10th: Reduce Consumption of Trans Fat

Studies by the FDA reveal that foods high in trans-fat have higher levels of C-reactive protein, a biomarker for inflammation in the body. Foods like cookies and crackers, margarines, and any products with partially or fully hydrogenated oils are some of the foods with high trans-fat content.

11th: Use Fruits and Spices to Sweeten Your Meals

Instead of using sugar and harmful ingredients to sweeten your meals, use fruits that can act as natural sweeteners such as berries, apples, apricot, cinnamon, turmeric, ginger, sage, cloves, thyme, and rosemary.

Now that we have laid down the rules, the next thing we will do is to put what we've learnt into perspective i.e. what foods you should eat and what you should avoid. The next chapter has a comprehensive list of foods to consume and foods to avoid while on this diet. Consider printing out the chapter so you can use it as a reference each time you need to cook or make shopping decisions. If you do, it will not be long before you get used to the diet and can quickly decipher foods which foods you should and should not buy.

Chapter 3:
Health Benefits of the Anti-Inflammatory Diet

Improved Brain Performance

Chronic inflammation may affect the brain and cause mental exhaustion. In turn, mental exhaustion may trigger feelings of depression, anxiety, and indecisiveness.

When you eat too much processed foods, bad fats, carbs and sugar, it may cause some blood sugar abnormalities that could cause insulin resistance. Insulin resistance may cause altered gastrointestinal function that may negatively affect normal brain function.

When you stop eating pro-inflammatory foods and start eating anti-inflammatory foods, it gives your brain a health boost because you would be eating anti-oxidant-rich foods that increase your brain function instead of impairing it.

Improved Skin Texture and Appearance

The skin is the largest organ in the body and as such, whatever you eat negatively or positively affects the skin. A poor diet may trigger skin inflammatory conditions. For instance, eating processed foods, sugar, and bad fats can cause leaky gut, something that forms from an imbalanced gut flora. Leaky gut could increase inflammation in the body and then cause skin problems like acne, itchiness, psoriasis, dull skin, and rosacea and skin rashes.

When you eliminate pro-inflammatory foods and introduce the foods you will be eating while on the anti-inflammatory diet, your skin appearance shall improve, so shall be your skin's texture with the resultant effect being a glowing and fresh looking skin.

Improved Weight Loss and Control of Cravings

Excessive food cravings are the reason why most people find it difficult to lose weight. The thing is; consumption of sugar and starch increases your cravings. Sugar cravings are not normal; it simply shows something is out of balance within your body system. Consuming excess sugars sets off a vicious cycle of food and sugar cravings that affects the chemicals in your brain. The more you continue consuming sugary foods, the worse the situation gets and the more your body becomes susceptible to inflammation.

The foods the anti-inflammatory diet advocates for help reduce cravings. Spices such as cinnamon, cloves, and cardamom have properties that help you control cravings. When you effectively reduce and control your cravings, you will lose weight because reduced cravings lead to a reduction in the calories you consume and eventually, reduced calorie consumption leads to weight loss.

An anti-inflammatory diet shall also see you eliminate many of the foods that make it difficult for you to lose weight. It also eliminates insulin and leptin resistance, which affects metabolism and promotes weight gain.

Reduction of Bloating

Foods like gluten and dairy products promote bloating. This is because of something called Dysbiosis. Dysbiosis refers to a situation where bad microorganisms overshadow good microorganisms. There should be a balance in the community of microorganisms in your gut. However, consumption of inflammatory foods promotes the growth of bad bacteria with the resultant effect being excessive bloating.

Dysbiosis can also occur when bacteria gets into the small intestines. Some anti-inflammatory foods have probiotics that increase the growth and spread of good bacteria that rectify and reverse the imbalance in your gut so you no longer feel bloated.

Prevents Autoimmunity

According to recent statistics, about 50 million Americans suffer from autoimmune disorders. Autoimmunity refers to a health condition where your immune system erroneously identifies your cells and tissues as harmful, and begins working against them. Inflammatory foods create antibodies that may trigger autoimmunity; hence, phasing out inflammatory foods and incorporating anti-inflammatory ones could help you stop consuming foods that may trigger autoimmune responses since most anti-inflammatory foods have detoxifying properties that help eliminate the antibodies before your immune system can start reacting.

Cures Adrenal Fatigue

Some of the most important hormones your body needs to be healthy include the Aldosterone and Cortisol. Cortisol controls and aids metabolism while aldosterone contributes to the regulation of blood pressure. The adrenal glands are responsible for producing these two hormones. Any malfunction of the adrenal glands affects the entire body system.

If your body becomes severely inflamed, something bound to happen when you consume excess amounts of refined carbs, adrenal fatigue may occur. Some symptoms of adrenal fatigue include depression, weight gain, anxiety, fatigue, inability to focus, excessive food cravings, burnouts, and difficulty getting out of bed.

Removing inflammatory foods from your diet can help boost adrenal system function and alleviate the symptoms of adrenal fatigue.

Alleviation of Allergies

Inflammatory foods may compromise your gut and make your body more susceptible to food allergies. The anti-inflammatory diet asks that you consume less of foods that may increase food allergies (such as food additives, fermented foods, processed meats, soy sauce, yeasty food, white wine, and beer).

One of the greatest things about the anti-inflammatory diet is that to derive these benefits, you need not do a complete overhaul of your regular diet. You simply need to incorporate beneficial foods and eliminate the harmful ones: no starvation, and no calorie counting. I believe you have realized just how easy it is to follow an anti-inflammatory diet. You can combine what you have learnt with several lifestyle changes for greater effectiveness. Some of the lifestyle changes you can embrace include:

- Reducing stress: Remember cortisol, the stress hormone, is highly inflammatory if it lingers for too long. Also, stress affects the adrenal glands negatively resulting to inflammatory responses if the problem sticks around for too long.

- Getting enough sleep: This will greatly help you to restore the much needed balance, which will provide a friendly environment for fighting inflammation effortlessly.

- Being physically active: This will help you to fight stress, enhance metabolism, protect your muscles, protect the heart and much more. Physical activity also helps to strengthen your immune system.

- Getting enough water: Water is very important in the process of fighting inflammation as it helps in the removal of toxins, improves digestion and enhances brain function.

Also, make sure to reduce your exposure to various toxins as these can easily trigger inflammatory responses. You can do that by giving up some bad habits that expose you to toxins like smoking, taking alcohol, drug use etc.

**********End of sample chapters**********

Anti – inflammatory Diet for beginners by Jonathan Smith

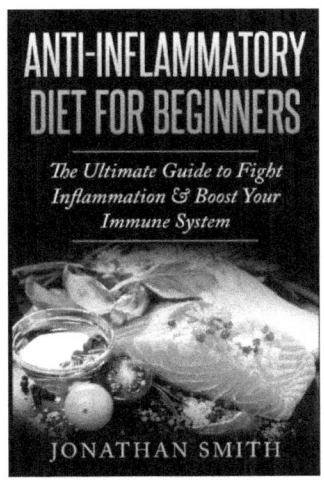

Bonus #2

Sample chapters of Anti – cancer Diet by Olivia Green

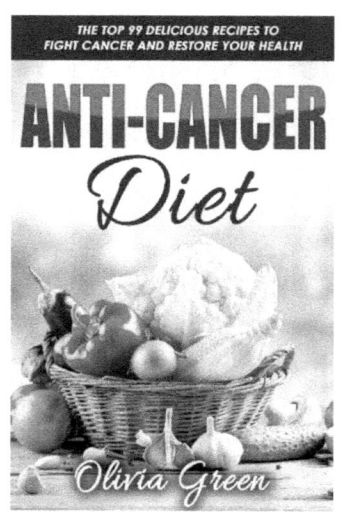

Chapter 1:
Role of Food in Tackling Cancer

What is cancer? To make it simple – "an abnormal growth." How does it happen? An uncontrolled cell division leads to tumor or abnormal cell growth i.e., when the tumor cells grow and divide beyond any control, they invade the tissues around the tumor and eventually spread to other body parts including your lymphatic systems and blood leading to painful or painless growth in the body. How do you avoid or control this? Consuming plenty of anti-cancer foods with antioxidants and natural anti-inflammatory phytonutrients can help reduce the risk of cancer.

Before discussing the anti-cancer diet chart, you need to understand and be very clear on your current food consumption and the dangerous food items that need to be completely avoided.

Food to avoid

Foods contributing to cancer usually include pesticides, preservatives, chemicals, animal products, artificial sweeteners, additives and dairy. It is a no brainer that we should be keeping away from these elements. However, we knowingly or unknowingly end up eating food laced with these products. Our fast food habits are the biggest cause of the consumption of these cancer-causing foods, which should be avoided at cost.

To be more specific, the following cancer causing foods must definitely be avoided from your regular diet

Processed meat
The meat you consume is full of hormones and preservatives to prolong shelf life and to improve taste. Processed meat should be left back on the shelf at the supermarket.

Red meat
It has already been proven that consumption of red meat is directly linked to a "high risk of cancer." Of course, I would not ask to completely avoid red meat but you can definitely lower the amount you consume.

Soda
Why drink it when you know it is loaded with sugar, artificial ingredients and calories that have no nutrition? Sadly, a lot of us are addicted to these sugary colas, which doesn't help your body in any way. You need to cut out sodas completely as soon as possible.

Fried / overly cooked food
Acrylamide, which is cancerous, is formed when the food is heated to a high temperature. Most food loses its nutrition when fried at a high temperature. Instead, try roasting your food.

Added sugar / artificial sweeteners
High consumption of added sugar can increase the risk of esophageal cancer, small intestine cancer, colon cancer and breast cancer.

Microwave popcorn
Chemicals in this popcorn can cause testicular, pancreatic and liver cancer. You can instead use popcorn kernels that are not dabbed in butter or any flavor and instead pop them in a wide bottomed pan with a bit of olive oil, salt and turmeric.

Processed food
Processed food usually contains dietary emulsifiers, which increase tumor formation, low-grade inflammation and colon carcinogenesis.

Cancer fighting food

Most of the plant-based food has phytonutrients that naturally prevent the human body from contracting various diseases.

Consciously including the below mentioned cancer fighting foods will reduce the risk of cancer in your life:

- Garlic
- Berries
- Tomatoes (Cooked)
- Cruciferous vegetables (Broccoli, Cabbage, Cauliflower)
- Green tea
- Whole grains
- Turmeric
- Leafy green vegetables (Spinach, Lettuce, Mustard greens, Collard greens, etc.)
- Grapes
- Beans
- Carrots
- Salads and green juices
- Unrefined oils

Cancer prevention tips

Your diet and its quality of life are linked to your health and its ability to prevent cancer. Apart from having a nutritional diet, there are few other things that are important to prevent cancer. Regular exercise, avoiding frequent medication, putting an end to smoking, reducing alcohol consumption, proper sleep and controlling your stress are the other things which needs to be on your "to-do" list.

Do check out the following and try implementing them:

- Have a fruit-rich diet to avoid lung and stomach cancer
- Add vegetables rich in carotenoids (carrots, sprouts, ripe tomatoes) to prevent larynx cancer, pharynx cancer, lung cancer and mouth cancer.
- Eat non-starchy vegetables (spinach, beans, broccoli) to avoid esophageal and stomach cancer
- Vitamin C rich foods (bell peppers, peas, leafy greens, berries, oranges,) can help avoid esophageal cancer
- Consume foods rich in lycopene (tomatoes, guava, watermelon,) to avoid prostate cancer

Focus on a healthy nutritious lifestyle to lead a stress free life. To ensure you follow your anti-cancer diet religiously, talk to your body, understand its needs, help your body with the cleansing and detoxifying process, drink loads of water, give enough Vitamin D to your body, eat organic and unprocessed food.

Chapter 2: Anti-Cancer Smoothie Recipes

Anti-Cancer Breakfast Smoothie

Broccoli and strawberries are excellent sources of anti-oxidants and vitamin C. Strawberries are having quercetin that destructs cancer cells.

Preparation time: 5 minutes

Number of servings: 1-2

Ingredients:

- 2 tablespoons hemp seeds
- 1 small ripe banana, sliced
- ¼ cup frozen or fresh pomegranate arils
- 2 cups salad greens or kale or spinach or collard greens
- 1 tablespoon cocoa powder
- ½ tablespoon ground chia seeds
- Juice of ½ lime
- 1 ½ cups filtered water
- ½ cup frozen strawberries
- ½ inch fresh ginger, sliced
- A handful fresh mint leaves
- 1 tablespoon flax meal
- ¼ cup frozen raw broccoli florets

Directions:

- If you are using kale or spinach or collard greens, then steam it for 5-6 minutes.
- Cool completely.
- Add hemp seeds and water into a blender and blend for 12-15 seconds.
- Add strawberries, banana and pomegranate and blend for another 12-15 seconds.
- Add cocoa, mint leaves, flax meal, broccoli, chia seeds, lime juice ginger and the greens that you are using. Blend for 30-40 seconds or until smooth. Add more water if you like a smoothie of thinner consistency.
- Pour into tall glass and serve with crushed ice right away.

Super Healthy Smoothie

Goji berries help in increasing the body's immunity and energy. They are high in carotenoids. All bright colored fruit and vegetables are high in carotenoids and are essential for building the immunity of the body.

Preparation time: 10 minutes

Number of servings: 1-2

Ingredients:

- 2 -3 tablespoons goji berries
- 20 raspberries
- 1 small avocado, peeled, pitted chopped
- ½ small beetroot, peeled, chopped
- 20 seedless red grapes
- 4 small broccoli florets
- 1 ½ cups coconut water or water
- 1 teaspoon olive oil

Directions:

- Add goji berries, raspberries, avocado, beetroot, grapes, broccoli, olive oil and coconut water into a blender and blend for 30-40 seconds or until smooth. Add more coconut water if you like your smoothie to be thinner in consistency.
- Pour into a tall glass and serve with crushed ice.

Green Smoothie

Spinach, romaine lettuce and kale are excellent sources of beta-carotene and vitamin C. Ginger is known to prevent cancer and inhibit tumor cell growth.

Preparation time: 10 minutes

Number of servings: 2

Ingredients:

- 2 medium bananas, sliced, frozen
- 2 cups spinach, torn
- 2 cups kale leaves, discard hard ribs and stem
- 2 cups celery, chopped
- 2 cups romaine lettuce, torn
- A handful mint leaves
- A handful fresh parsley
- 2 inch piece fresh ginger, sliced
- 2 medium cucumbers, chopped
- 2 small pear or Granny Smith apple, cored, chopped, peel if desired
- 1 teaspoon ground cinnamon
- 4 tablespoons lemon juice
- 1 tablespoon chia seeds
- A pinch cayenne pepper
- 2 cups coconut water or water
- Natural sweetener like stevia or honey (optional), to

Directions:

- Add banana, spinach, kale, celery, lettuce, mint parsley, ginger, cucumber, pear or apple, cinnamon,

lemon juice, chia seeds, cayenne pepper, coconut water and sweetener if using into a blender and blend until smooth.
- Add more coconut water if you desire a smoothie of thinner consistency.
- Pour into a tall glass and serve with crushed ice.

Orange Wheatgrass Smoothie

Wheat grass is known to prevent cancer. It is loaded with vitamins, minerals is an anti-oxidant.

Preparation time: 5 minutes

Number of servings: 2

Ingredients:

- ½ cup water or coconut water
- ½ cup fresh wheatgrass or ½ teaspoon wheatgrass powder
- 1 banana, peeled, sliced, frozen
- 1 cup almond milk or soy milk
- 2 oranges or 4 tangerines, peeled (the thin membrane from the segments as well), deseeded
- 1 cup ice

Directions:

- Add the ingredients into a blender in the order mentioned – coconut water, almond milk, wheat grass, tangerine, banana and ice.
- Blend for 30-40 seconds or until smooth. Add more coconut water if you want a smoothie of thinner consistency.
- Pour into tall glasses and serve.

Red Smoothie

Turmeric contains curcumin, which is anti-cancerous. It is also known to reduce the size of tumors.

Preparation time: 5 minutes

Number of servings: 2

Ingredients:

- 1 banana, sliced, frozen
- 4 stalks kale, discard hard stems and ribs, torn
- 1 inch fresh ginger, peeled, sliced
- ½ teaspoon turmeric powder
- 1 teaspoon organic coconut oil
- 2 teaspoons black nigella seeds
- ¼ cup raspberries
- 4 strawberries, chopped
- 2 carrots, chopped
- 2 cups red cabbage, shredded
- A pinch black pepper
- 2 teaspoons chia seeds
- 2 cups almond milk
- Ice cubes, as required

Directions:

- Add banana, kale, ginger, turmeric powder, coconut oil, nigella seeds, raspberries, strawberries, carrots, red cabbage, pepper, chia seeds, almond milk and ice cubes into a blender.

- Blend for 30-40 seconds or until smooth. Add more almond milk if you like a smoothie of thinner consistency.
- Pour into tall glasses and serve.

Green Super Foods Smoothie

Probiotic foods stop the growth of tumors and help in cell growth. Chia seeds and wheatgrass powder are anti-cancerous.

Preparation time: 10 minutes

Number of servings: 3-4

Ingredients:

- 2 green tea bags
- 1 cup unfiltered apple juice
- 2 medium bananas, sliced
- 4 tablespoons lemon juice
- 4 teaspoons wheatgrass powder
- 4 cups frozen pineapple chunks, unsweetened
- 2 cups hot water
- 1 teaspoon probiotic powder
- 6 tablespoons sprouted chia seed powder
- 2 cups firmly packed baby spinach
- 2 tablespoons hemp seed protein powder
- A pinch Celtic sea salt

Directions:

- Drop the tea bags in hot water for a minute. Discard the tea bags and cool completely.
- Pour the brewed tea into a blender. Add apple juice, banana, lemon juice, wheatgrass powder, pineapple, probiotic powder, chia seed powder, spinach, hemp seed powder and salt into a blender.

- Blend for 30-40 seconds or until smooth. Add more water if you like a smoothie of thinner consistency.
- Pour into tall glasses and serve with crushed ice.

Chapter 3:
Anti-Cancer Juice Recipes

Tomato Juice

Tomatoes help in preventing the DNA in the cells from getting damaged. Tomatoes are high in lycopene. Garlic and ginger help in preventing cancer.

Preparation time: 10 minutes

Number of servings: 2

Ingredients:

- 8 tomatoes, chopped into chunks
- 1 bell pepper, deseeded, chopped into chunks
- 4 stalks celery, chopped into pieces
- 1 small bunch parsley
- 1 small bunch cilantro
- 2 inch piece fresh ginger, peeled, sliced
- 4 tablespoons lemon juice
- 2 cloves garlic, peeled

Directions:

- Juice together tomatoes, bell pepper, celery, parsley, and cilantro, and ginger, garlic and lemon juice in a juicer.
- Alternately, you can add all the ingredients into a blender and blend until smooth.

- Strain if desired.
- Pour into tall glasses and serve with crushed ice.

Sunrise Juice

Bright colored fruit and vegetables are high in vitamin C and beta-carotene.

Preparation time: 10 minutes

Number of servings: 2

Ingredients:

- 2 medium sized pink grapefruit, peeled, deseeded
- 2 apples, cored, sliced
- 8 medium carrots, chopped
- 2 inch piece ginger, sliced
- Juice of a lemon

Directions:

- Juice together grapefruit, apples, carrots and ginger into a juicer. Add lemon juice and stir.
- Alternately, you can add the ingredients into a blender and blend until smooth.
- Strain if desired.
- Pour into tall glasses. Add lemon juice and stir.
- Serve with ice.

Vibrant Green Ginger Tonic

This green juice is full of antioxidants, vitamins and minerals. Kale celery and parsley contain lots of it.

Preparation time: 10 minutes

Number of servings: 2

Ingredients:

- Juice of 2 lemons
- 3 inch piece of ginger, peeled, chopped
- A pinch of salt
- 2 green apples, cored, sliced
- 10 stalks of celery, chopped
- 10 kale leaves, discard hard stems and ribs, torn
- 2 handfuls parsley
- Lemon zest to garnish

Directions:

- Juice together ginger, apple, celery, kale and parsley in a juicer
- Alternately, you can add the ingredients into a blender and blend until smooth.
- Strain if desired.
- Pour into tall glasses. Add lemon juice and stir.
- Garnish with lemon zest.
- Sprinkle with a pinch of salt and cayenne pepper if you like it spicy. Serve with ice cubes.

Tornado Juice

Citrus fruit is high in vitamin C. Tomatoes have lycopene.

Preparation time: 12-15 minutes

Number of servings: 2

Ingredients:

- 2 oranges, peeled, separated into segments
- ½ lemon, peeled, deseeded
- 2 medium carrots, chopped
- 4 stalks celery, chopped
- 2 cucumbers, chopped
- 2 apples, cored, chopped
- 2 inches fresh ginger, sliced
- 1 cup spinach
- 2 cups cherry tomatoes

Directions:

- Juice together oranges, lemon, carrots, celery, cucumbers, apples, ginger, spinach and cherry tomatoes in a juicer.
- Alternately, you can add the ingredients into a blender and blend until smooth.
- Strain if desired.
- Pour into tall glasses.
- You can either have it plain or even hot. It tastes good with ice too.

Papaya Pineapple Blast

Bright colored fruit is oozing with phytochemicals. Cashew nuts are full of healthy fatty acids. This juice is full of vitamin C that keeps your immunity strong.

Preparation time: 15 minutes

Number of servings: 2

Ingredients:

- 1 cup pomegranate arils
- 1 cup ripe papaya chunks
- 1 cup pineapple chunks
- 6 strawberries, chopped
- 2 cups mixed greens
- 10 cashew nuts
- 1 teaspoon coconut oil
- 2 cups coconut water

Directions:

- Juice together pomegranate arils, papaya, pineapple, strawberries, mixed greens, cashew nuts, coconut oil and coconut water in a juicer.
- Alternately, you can add the ingredients into a blender and blend until smooth.
- Strain if desired.
- Pour into tall glasses.
- Serve with crushed ice.

Purple Power Juice

Red cabbage is a cruciferous vegetable that is anti-cancerous. Purple grapes are high in resveratrol, which is anti-cancerous.

Preparation time: 10 minutes

Number of servings: 2

Ingredients:

- 2 cucumbers, chopped
- 4 stalks celery, chopped
- 2 Granny Smith apples, cored, chopped
- 2 cups purple grapes
- 2 inch piece fresh ginger, chopped
- 2 carrots, chopped
- 2 beets, sliced
- Greens of 2 beets, chopped
- 1 small red cabbage, cut into wedges

Directions:

- Add cucumber, celery, apples, grapes, ginger, carrots, beets, beet greens and cabbage into a blender and blend until smooth.
- Strain if desired.
- Alternately, juice together in a juicer.
- Pour into tall glasses and serve with ice.

Chapter 4:
Anti-Cancer Breakfast Recipes

Quinoa Porridge

Quinoa is rich in protein and all the essential amino acids. Sugar is well utilized in the body with cinnamon. The sugar quickly goes from the blood into the cells to use as energy.

Preparation time: 10 minutes

Number of servings: 6

Ingredients:

- 2 cups quinoa, rinsed
- 4 cups water
- 6 teaspoons ground cinnamon
- 1 cup dried cranberries or currants
- 1 cup hemp hearts
- Maple syrup or honey to taste
- 2 cups coconut milk
- 4 cups water
- 3 teaspoons ground ginger
- 4 apples, cored, chopped
- 1 cup walnuts, chopped

Directions:

- Add quinoa, water, ginger, cinnamon, coconut milk, cranberries and apples into a heavy bottomed pan.
- Place the pan over medium heat. Bring to the boil.

- Lower heat and cover with a lid. Simmer until quinoa is cooked and all the water is dry.
- Divide into bowls. Sprinkle walnuts and hemp hearts. Top with honey or maple syrup and serve.

Pumpkin-Papaya Acai Bowl

Pumpkin is low in calories. It is high in potassium, fiber, phytoestrogens and beta-carotene and protects the body against free radicals, which is the major cause for cancer.

Preparation time: 10 minutes

Number of servings: 6

Ingredients:

For the acai bowl:

- 1 cup papaya, chopped into chunks
- 1 cup canned pumpkin
- 2 medium bananas, sliced
- 2 frozen acai smoothie pack, unsweetened
- 1 tablespoon ground cinnamon
- 1 tablespoon pumpkin pie spice
- 2 tablespoons maca powder
- 2 cups almond milk

To serve:

- 1 cup goji berries
- ½ cup cashews, chopped, toasted
- A few slices papaya
- A few slices banana
- ½ cup pomegranate seeds
- ½ cup granola

Directions:

- Add papaya, pumpkin, banana, acai smoothie pack, cinnamon, pumpkin pie spice, maca powder and

almond milk into the blender and blend until smooth. Pour into 6 serving bowls. Chill if desired.
- Add papaya and banana slices and pomegranate seeds and stir.
- Sprinkle goji berries, cashews and granola on top and serve right away.

Veggie Egg Muffins

Turmeric has curcumin, which is an anti-oxidant and promotes apoptosis (cancer cells are killed). Spinach and bright colored bell peppers are great anti-cancer foods.

Preparation time: 15 minutes

Number of servings: 6

Ingredients:

- 6 eggs
- 1 large tomato, chopped
- ½ teaspoon turmeric powder
- 1 large onion, chopped
- 2 cloves garlic, minced
- 1 orange or red bell pepper, chopped
- ½ cup spinach, chopped
- Salt and Pepper as per taste
- A handful fresh basil, chopped

Directions:

- Grease 6 muffin cups. Place disposable liners in them.
- Add eggs and coconut milk in a medium bowl and whisk the contents well. Add turmeric, salt and pepper and whisk well.
- Add onion, bell pepper, spinach and tomatoes and stir.
- Spoon into the muffin cups. Fill up to ¾.
- Bake in a preheated oven at 350º F for 15 minutes or until set. A toothpick when inserted in the center should come out clean.
- Let it remain in the oven for 10 minutes.

- Remove from the oven and cool for a while. Run a knife around the edges to loosen the muffins. Invert on to a plate.
- Serve warm.

Cauliflower Pancakes

Eggs contain choline and it reduces the risk of cancer especially breast cancer. Cauliflower is a cruciferous vegetable that is highly beneficial in fighting cancer.

Preparation time: 10 minutes

Number of servings: 3

Ingredients:

- 1 large head cauliflower, broken into florets
- 3 tablespoons flat leaf parsley, chopped
- 3 eggs
- ¾ cup leeks, cleaned, chopped
- ¾ cup almond flour
- 2 cups smoked gouda cheese, shredded (optional)
- Salt to taste
- Pepper powder to taste
- 4-5 tablespoons coconut oil
- Eggs for serving

Directions:

- Place cauliflower florets in the food processor bowl and pulse until you get rice like texture. Alternately you can grate it. Transfer into a bowl.
- Place a skillet over low heat and add ½ tablespoon oil. When the oil is heated, add leeks and sauté until translucent.
- Add garlic and sauté for a few seconds until fragrant. Remove from heat and transfer into the bowl of cauliflower. Mix well.

- Add parsley, salt, pepper, almond flour, 3 eggs and Gouda cheese if using. Mix until well combined.
- Place a nonstick pan over low heat and add ½ teaspoon oil. When oil is heated, add about a heaping tablespoonful of cauliflower mixture on the pan and spread a little using the back of a spoon.
- Cook until the underside is golden brown. Flip sides and cook the other side too.
- Remove on to a serving platter.
- Repeat step 5 and 6 to make the remaining pancakes
- Cook eggs sunny side up. Serve pancakes with eggs.

Power up Breakfast Burrito

Low fat cheese helps in reducing the risk of colon cancer. Spinach or kale is anti-cancerous. Berries are high in anti-oxidants.

Preparation time: 10 minutes

Number of servings: 4

Ingredients:

- 4 teaspoons olive oil
- 2 cups fresh spinach or kale, shredded
- 3-4 tablespoons skim milk
- 4 whole wheat tortillas
- 1 medium red onion, chopped (optional)
- 4 eggs
- 4 ounces low fat mozzarella cheese, shredded
- Berries to serve
- Salt to taste
- Pepper to taste

Directions:

- Place a skillet over low heat and add oil. When the oil is heated, add onion and sauté until translucent.
- Add spinach and sauté until it turns bright green in color.
- Meanwhile, add eggs and milk into a bowl. Whisk well.
- Pour into the skillet along with mozzarella. Stir frequently until the eggs are scrambled and cooked. Season with salt and pepper

- Warm the tortillas following the instructions on the package.
- Spread the tortillas on a serving platter. Divide the mixture among the 4 tortillas. Do not place filling on the sides.
- Fold the bottom of the tortilla. Fold the sides together. Roll the tortillas.
- Wrap in paper towels.
- Serve with berries of your choice.

Green Tea-Scented Quinoa with Corn

Green tea has catechins, which are antioxidants that are highly anti-cancerous, and destroys the cancer cells. Quinoa, broccoli sprouts and carrots are high in anti-oxidants.

Preparation time: 14 minutes

Number of servings: 2

Ingredients:

- ½ cup quinoa, rinsed
- Salt to taste
- 2 tablespoons fresh or frozen corn kernels
- 1 clove garlic, minced
- 1 teaspoon lemon juice
- 2 sprigs parsley, chopped
- 1 teaspoon flaxseed oil
- Fistful broccoli sprouts
- 1 cup lightly brewed green tea
- 14 cup scallion, finely chopped
- ¼ cup carrot, finely chopped

Directions:

- Add quinoa and green tea into a saucepan. Place the saucepan over medium heat. Bring to the boil.
- Add corn, scallion, salt, garlic and carrot and stir.
- Lower heat and cover with a lid. Simmer until dry.
- Add parsley, lemon juice and flaxseed oil and loosen with a fork.
- Garnish with broccoli sprouts and serve.

Chapter 5: Anti-cancer Snack Recipes

Sweet Potato Fries

Sweet potatoes have loads of beta-carotene, fiber, vitamin C etc. They reduce the risk of lung cancer, colon cancer, breast cancer and stomach cancer.

Preparation time: 10 minutes

Number of servings: 4

Ingredients:

- 4 medium sweet potatoes, scrubbed or peeled, sliced into julienne strips
- 1 teaspoon chili powder
- 1 teaspoon pepper powder
- 1 teaspoon ground cumin
- ½ teaspoon cayenne pepper
- Sea salt to taste
- 2 tablespoons extra virgin olive oil

Directions:

- Add sweet potatoes, chili powder, cumin, pepper, and cayenne pepper, salt into a bowl and toss well.
- Drizzle oil on top and toss well.
- Transfer on to a greased baking sheet and spread it in a single layer.

- Bake in a preheated oven 425° F for about 30 minutes or until the top is light brown in color. It should be tender inside and crisp outside. Turn the sweet potatoes half way through baking.
- Serve hot with a dip of your choice.

Cheese Balls

Goat's cheese and chia seeds are nutrient dense. Chia seeds and almonds are high in fiber and omega– 3 fatty acids.

Preparation time: 15 minutes

Number of servings: 6 (3 balls each)

Ingredients:

- 4 ounces plain almond milk cream cheese
- 4 ounces goat's cheese
- ¼ teaspoon garlic, minced
- A handful fresh cilantro, finely chopped
- ¼ cup roasted, salted almonds, chopped
- 4 teaspoons chia seeds
- Pepper powder to taste
- Salt to taste

Directions:

- Add goat's cheese and cream cheese into a bowl.
- Beat with an electric mixer on medium speed until smooth.
- Add cilantro, salt, pepper and garlic and mix. Place the bowl in the freezer for 15 minutes.
- Add nuts into the food processor bowl and pulse until fine. Transfer into a bowl. Add chia seeds and mix.
- Divide the mixture into 18 equal portions and shape into balls.
- Dredge the balls in the nut mixture. Place in an airtight container and refrigerate until use.
- Serve with a dip of your choice.

Spinach Rolls with Ricotta & Pistachios

Spinach is high in vitamin C and A. These are anti-bacterial and anti-viral and have the capability to prevent formation of tumors.

Preparation time: 10 minutes

Number of servings: 8

Ingredients:

- 4 tablespoons extra virgin olive oil, divided
- 18 ounces fresh spinach, rinsed, discard tough stems, finely chopped
- 14 ounces part skim ricotta
- ½ cup low fat parmesan cheese, grated, divided
- 1 teaspoon ground nutmeg
- 8 whole wheat lasagna sheets, cook according to the instructions on the package
- 2 cups pistachio nuts, finely chopped
- Salt to taste

Directions:

- Place a skillet over low heat and add half the oil. When the oil is heated, add spinach and salt and sauté until the spinach wilts.
- Remove from heat and cool completely. Transfer into a bowl.
- Add ricotta, half the Parmesan, nutmeg, and pistachio nuts and salt and set aside.
- Dry the cooked lasagna sheets with paper towels. Place a lasagna sheet on your countertop.

- Spread the cheese mixture over it. Roll and set aside.
- Repeat with the remaining mixture and lasagna sheets.
- Cut into slices of about 1-2 inches. Drizzle the remaining oil over it and sprinkle the remaining cheese on top and serve.
- If you like the cheese melted, microwave on high for a few seconds until the cheese melts and serve.

Vegan Spinach Balls

Spinach is an antioxidant and detoxifies your body.

Preparation time: 5 minutes

Number of servings: 10

Ingredients:

- 1 ½ cups fresh spinach
- ½ cup almonds
- ¼ cup cashews
- 1 ½ tablespoons olive oil
- ½ tablespoon chia seeds or flax seeds mixed with 1 ½ tablespoons water (egg replacer)
- ¼ cup oats
- ¼ teaspoon salt
- 1 small onion, quartered

Directions:

- Place a sheet of parchment paper on a baking sheet.
- Add spinach, almonds, cashews, oil, chia mixture, oats, salt and onions into the food processor bowl. Pulse until coarse in texture.
- Transfer into a bowl.
- Divide the mixture into 1-tablespoon portions and shape into balls.
- Place on the prepared baking sheet.
- Bake in a preheated oven 350° F for about 30 minutes or until light brown in color.
- Remove from the oven and cool for a while.
- Serve warm with a dip of your choice.

Lean Meatballs with Teriyaki Sauce

Sesame seeds are dense in nutrients. They are high in calcium and vitamin E. Honey is anti-inflammatory and anti-bacterial. It is anti-cancer.

Preparation time: 20 minutes

Number of servings: 8

Ingredients:

For teriyaki sauce:

- 4 tablespoons honey
- 5 tablespoons light soy sauce or tamari
- 4 tablespoons rice wine vinegar

For meatballs:

- 2 pounds lean ground beef or turkey
- 4 slices whole wheat bread, discard the sides
- 1 onion, minced
- 2 green onions, chopped, for garnishing
- ½ cup milk
- 2 tablespoons sesame seeds, toasted + extra for garnishing
- Salt to taste
- Pepper powder to taste
- 2 tablespoons sesame oil
- ¼ cup olive oil
- 2 eggs

Directions:

- To make teriyaki sauce: Mix together in a bowl, soy sauce, honey and rice wine vinegar and set aside.
- To make meatballs: Place bread slices in a bowl. Pour milk over it. Set aside for a few minutes and then squeeze the bread to drain off excess milk.
- Mix together in a large bowl the rest of the ingredients except olive oil. Add bread and mix well using your hands.
- Clean your hands and moisten if required.
- Make small balls of the mixture and set aside.
- Place a nonstick skillet over low heat and add 3 tablespoons of olive oil. When the oil is heated, add the meatballs and cook until brown on all the sides. Cook in batches if required.
- Add teriyaki sauce and mix well. Heat thoroughly.
- Garnish with green onions and sesame seeds. Insert toothpicks on the meatballs and serve immediately.

Quinoa Chia Seed Protein Bars

Quinoa suppresses the growth of cancer cells. They are high in protein and contain all the 9 essential amino acids. It is high in fiber, vitamin and minerals. Almonds are high in fiber and helps in building a strong immune system.

Preparation time: 5 minutes

Number of servings: 6

Ingredients:

- ¼ cup dry quinoa
- 1 tablespoon ground flax seeds
- A pinch Himalayan salt
- ½ teaspoon ground cardamom
- ½ teaspoon ground cinnamon
- 2 tablespoons honey
- ¼ cup almond butter
- ¼ cup chia seeds
- ½ cup rolled oats
- ¼ cup almonds, chopped
- 2 tablespoons brown rice syrup

Directions:

- Add almond butter, honey and brown rice syrup into a microwave safe bowl. Microwave on High for 40-50 seconds or until it melts. Mix well.
- Add quinoa, flaxseeds, salt, spices, chia seeds, oats and almonds into a bowl and stir.
- Transfer the almond butter mix into it. Mix well.

- Place rack in the middle of the oven
- Line a baking dish with butter paper. Transfer the mixture in the dish. Spread it evenly with a spatula.
- Bake in a preheated oven 350° F for about 15 minutes.
- Cool for 10-15 minutes. Remove the baked bar along with the parchment paper and cool on a wire rack.
- Cut into 6 equal squares and serve.

********End of sample chapters********

[Anti – cancer Diet by Olivia Green](#)

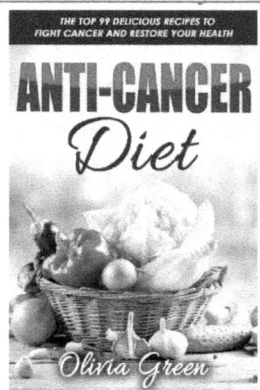

Thanks again for purchasing this book. We hope you enjoy it

Don't forget to claim your gift!

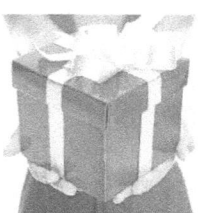

http://bit.ly/VBonus1

www.ingramcontent.com/pod-product-compliance
Lightning Source LLC
Chambersburg PA
CBHW050306230526
45471CB00005B/2050